Healing Honey For Beginners

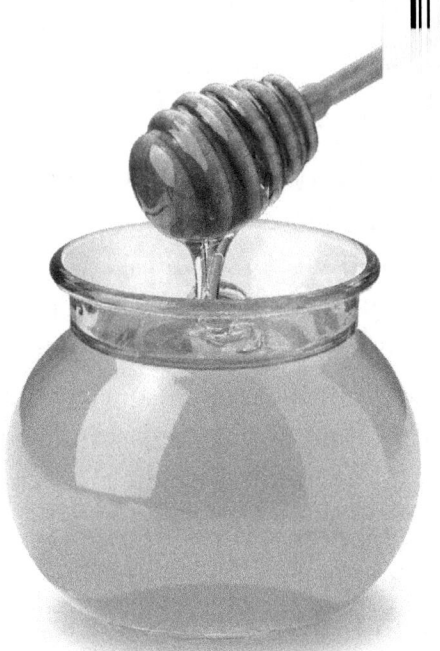

How To Use Honey To Cure, Beautify And Heal

Disclaimer

This book is intended to be a general guide, to raise awareness, and to help people make informed decisions in the context of their own personal circumstance. As everybody's circumstances are different, so are the remedies you should seek. While many of the recommendations in this book can be applied by almost anybody regardless of their conditions they are not intended to and should not be relied upon to replace personal medical advice.

The author accepts no responsibility for any loss or injury, be it personal or financial, as a result for the use or misuse of the information in this book. If you have any doubts or concerns after reading this book, please speak to a doctor or other qualified person before taking any actions.

From The Author

Thank you for taking the time to read this book. As an author, I understand the importance of creating books which my readers will find both enjoyable and informative. If you have the time and feel generous, please don't hesitate to leave an honest review of this book.........Dr Brad Turner.

Contents

Introduction

The jar of honey is a frequently seen item on our breakfast table. My kids just love to eat bread, honey, and butter. They never get tired of honey and it is a daily routine. Honey reminds them of nothing else but sweetness, and of course the bees!

Anyone would be aware of where honey comes from, and interestingly the honey bees visit more than 2 million flowers and fly about 55,000 miles to make one pound of honey. Surprised? The honey bees have been on this job for more than 10-20 million years and an average honey bee worker makes about 1/12 teaspoon of honey in their lifetime. I am sure only a few would realize that honey bees are the only insects that produce food for us. So a jar of honey costs more than money, it is a lot of hard work, effort, and a labour of love for humans. It is a pity that a honey bee will work herself to death just after about three weeks.

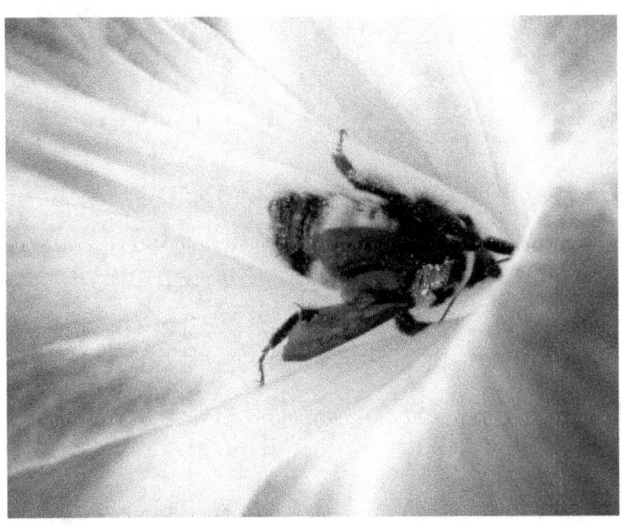

"If the bee disappears from the surface of the earth, man would have no more than four years to live?" - **Albert Einstein**

To go into more facts – Honey is made by honey bees using nectar from flowers. Thereafter the honey is collected by beekeepers for our consumption.

The Teeny-Weeny Workers

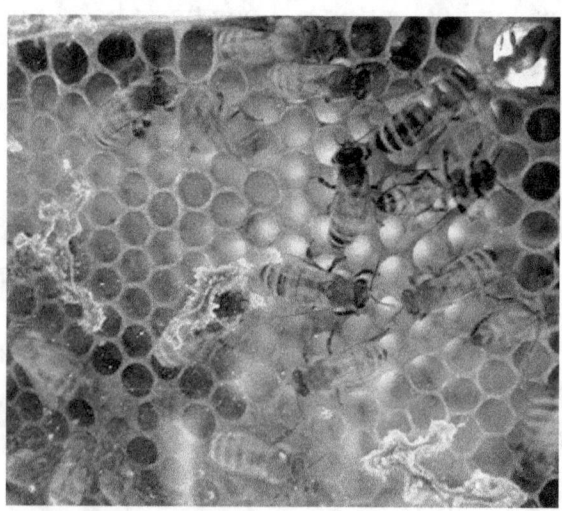

Different honey bees perform different jobs. The honey bees collect pollen and nectar from flowers when they are in full bloom. They use their long, tube-like tongues to drink the nectar and then they store it in their crop or stomachs. Thereafter it is taken to the bee hives. The stomach is only for storing purposes and within half an hour's time the nectar is processed where the enzyme called invertase converts the nectar into honey. Nectar consists of Sucrose and water. The bees take the nectar to the bee hives where they drop the honey into tiny hexagonal wax cells. The bees need to work hard to fill these tiny cells, as it can take in a huge load, and the process is repeated until the cells are full.

The job is not yet completed as the honey is wet and damp. Their next task is to fan their tiny wings, which helps the liquid to evaporate and thicken the honey. When done, the tiny cells are sealed with a wax which helps the honey to be kept clean. Then the bees move on to the next comb which stands empty and the busy bees start their jobs all over again.

To make one single teaspoonful of honey at least about 8 bees need to put in all their efforts and it takes them a lifetime to complete these tasks.

The honey collected is used during winter times when there are no flowers in bloom. However, a hive requires only a little portion of honey for their survival and the extra honey is harvested by beekeepers. They extract the liquid honey by removing the wax cap using a blunt knife and placing the bee hives in a centrifuge to get the honey out of the combs. Most often the beekeepers replace the empty comb by placing them back into the beehives for refilling. This eases the life of the bees as there is no requirement for them to re-build the combs. Some others use this to make candles by melting the wax.

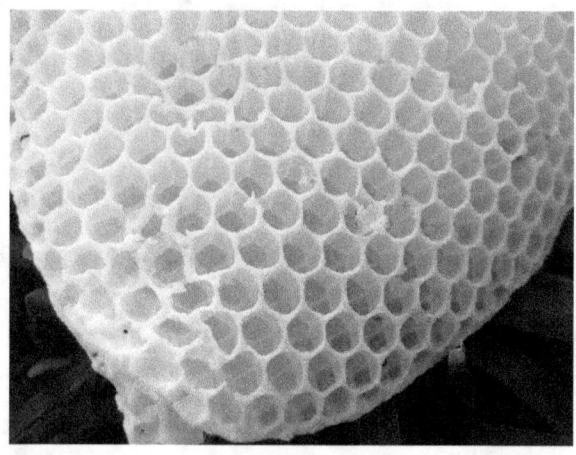

Thankfully, the bees store more than they ever need and we can pinch some of theirs for our use.

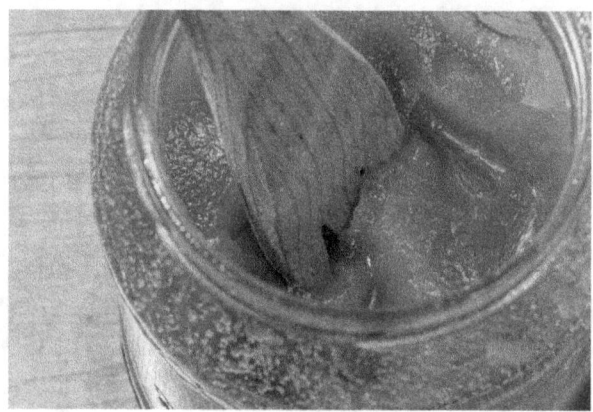

FACT
The tiny bee's brain is the size of a sesame seed and is oval shaped. Interestingly, the bee has a remarkable capacity to learn and remember things. They are able to solve complex calculations on distance and hunting efficiency.

Chapter 1

The History Of Honey & Humans

Honey has been in existence for many years, with humans hunting for honey over 8,000 years ago. A cave painting in Valencia, Spain depicts two honey hunters looking for honey and a honeycomb from a wild bee nest. However, fossils of honey bees date back to about 150M years, which goes on to say that honey would have played a vital role in history due to its nutrients and many uses. It is also said that honey was man's first source of sweetener until cane sugar came into the scene.

The earliest records of honey trace back 4,700 to 5,500 years ago to Georgia, where honey remains were found on the inner surface of a few clay vessels uncovered in an ancient tomb. During that era, people in Georgia packed honey to take for their journeys into the afterlife.

Honey was found to be effective for a variety of reasons and people of different cultures had consumed the liquid for different purposes based on their beliefs and customs.

Around the World!
In ancient Egypt, honey was used as a sweetener for preparing food and for medicinal reasons. Ancient Egyptians used honey for religious purposes, offering honey to their fertility God and also used the liquid for embalming the dead. The bee was a common royal symbol used by

Egyptians in the early days and was said to be favored by many a Pharaoh.

Past records of Vedas and Ayurveda indicate that in ancient India, honey was used for its spiritual and therapeutic purposes and the usage dates back to over 4,000 years ago.
The Greeks believed honey to be a healing medicine and was a common item used in their food with many Greek recipe books containing dishes made with honey.

The Romans used honey as an offering to the Gods and for cooking. It is also said that during the Roman Empire, beekeeping was a thriving home industry.

In the absence of sugar, honey played an important role in Europe until the Renaissance. When sugar was introduced, the demand for honey came down and usage became less.
Honey and beeswax demand increased to a certain extent when Christians started lighting candles for church services.

Bees were used in many emblems
Bees were thought to be important and have special powers. This was proven by the fact that the bee metaphor was used in many instances by the royalty, political leaders, and for religious purposes.

Chapter 2

The Main Differences Between The Honey And Cane Sugar

Honey Vs Sugar – Which is better?

If one is to ask which is better – Honey or Sugar, it will get you thinking, as most of us will use these commonly available ingredients without thinking of the value additions. After all, both honey and sugar are carbohydrate, calorie packed sweeteners.

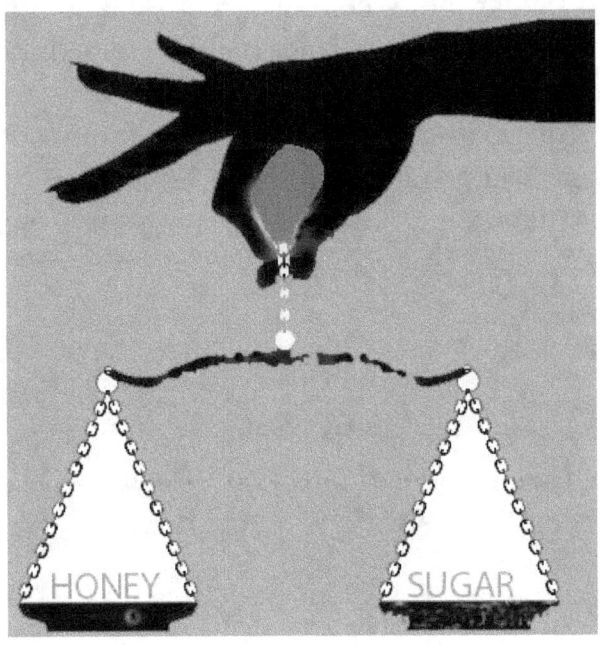

Similarities and Differences

Honey is nature's gift to mankind while sugar is a substance extracted from various plants, especially sugar cane and sugar beet.

Honey goes through only one processing step - the honey is heated to prevent crystallization and yeast fermentation occurring during storage. Honey contains antimicrobial and antioxidant properties which are not found in table sugar. Sugar is highly processed and in the production of table sugar, the process destroys all natural minerals, vitamins, enzymes, and almost all healthy components.

Honey and Sugar both contain fructose and glucose and carry the same relative sweetness. The formation is slightly different in sugar, as glucose and fructose are bound together to form sucrose. Sucrose, which comes from sugar cane, is commonly known as table sugar. In honey, the formation is different, as glucose and fructose remain separate units.

Sweeter - Which?

Fructose is sweeter than Glucose. This is the reason so much fructose is piled into our food today. Fructose converts into energy at a lesser pace than glucose, which means food containing fructose converts to fat more easily. Definitely a worrying factor for the weight watcher!

Bloodstream

Sucrose is not digested in the stomach due to its disaccharide composition – glucose-fructose structure. Once sucrose reaches the small intestine, the liver utilizes a few enzymes to convert the particles into glucose, which then enter the main bloodstream.

With honey it is a different story; the enzymes which are inserted into the nectar by the honey bees separate the sucrose into two units - fructose and glucose. These sugars are easily digested and directly absorbed into the bloodstream.

Calories
Calories play an important role in our lives today. Almost everyone is watching their calories nowadays and they are very conscious about their diets and workouts.

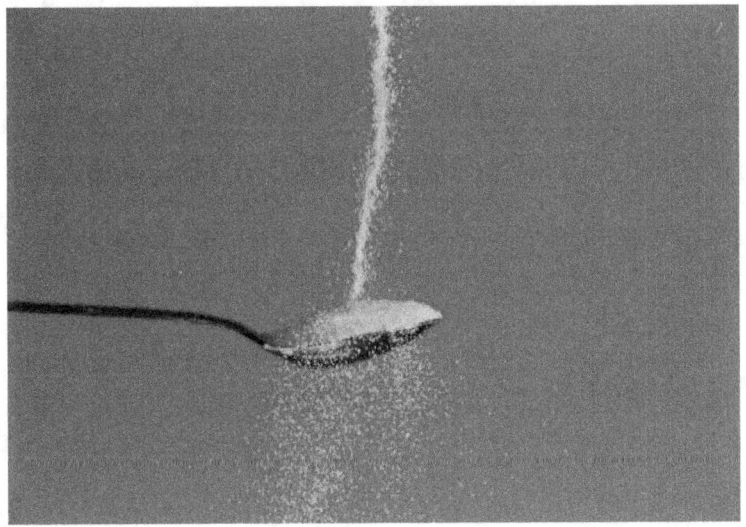

One teaspoon of sugar contains 16 calories while one teaspoon of honey contains 22 calories. In simple terms, honey has more calories. Since honey is sweeter, one needs to use only a lesser quantity of honey, which means a person will consume fewer calories. This is the reason honey has a higher density and weight against sugar.

GI

How carbohydrates deal with glucose in the bloodstream is measured by the glycemic index (GI). Honey contains a lower GI than sugar and research indicates that foods with lower GI lead to a relatively small increase in blood glucose. This means honey carries reduced risk of coronary heart disease, Type 2 Diabetes, and will not induce you to overeat.

Well, these are a few good reasons to invest in a pot of honey, although it is more costly than a packet of sugar!

FACT
Worker bees are all females and they work very hard.

Chapter 3

The Various Honey Varieties

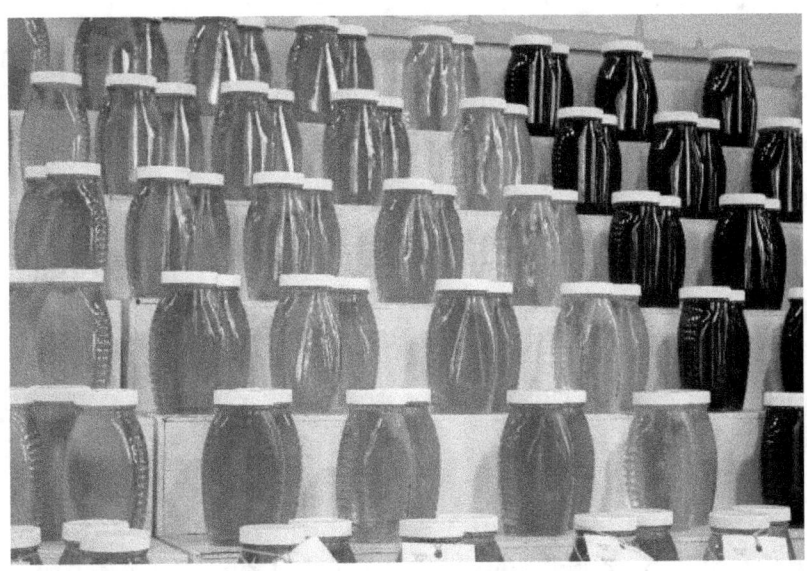

There are plenty of varieties of honey available in the market. If you look around a supermarket, you are likely to see enough and more bottles and jars of honey coming from all over the world.

The Difference?
Varieties mainly depend on the nectar source – in other words, the source of blossoms from where the bees collect pollen to make honey. Honey bees extract the nectar from different blooms; no wonder in the US alone it is said that there are more than 300 unique types of honey available in the market.

The colors, flavor, and aroma differ from one variety of honey to another. The colors can come in dark brown to colorless, the flavors from mild to bold, and odor most often is distinctive to the flower.

It is usually found that light colored honey is milder while dark colored honey is stronger. The honey from the same flower blooming in different locations will produce different nectar depending on the weather conditions of the area.

Honey is produced in most countries of the world, but certain types of honey are unique to a few regions. While there are different types of honey available, most honey supplied in bulk is blended to create the best honey - with a unique taste and flavor.

In this book, you will find a few common varieties of honey, as there will be hardly any space left if one is to list out all the existing varieties around the world.

Acacia

Acacia honey is very light in color and comes from the Black Locust or false Acacia tree. It has a very mild floral flavor and has a hint of vanilla taste. This is a very popular type of honey and it mixes well with beverages and cheese.

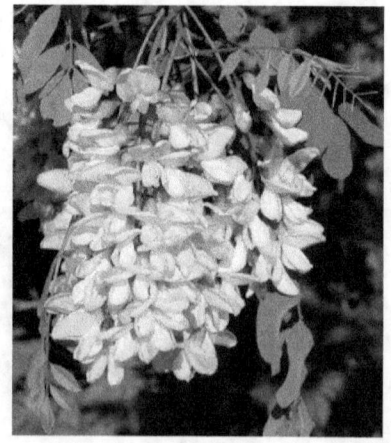

Acacia honey rarely crystallizes due to its high fructose content and is often used for cooking purposes.

Alfalfa
This honey comes from purple flowers which are common to the Western States. It is white or extra light amber in color with a very mild flavor and aroma. This variety is used often as a table honey in day to day life.

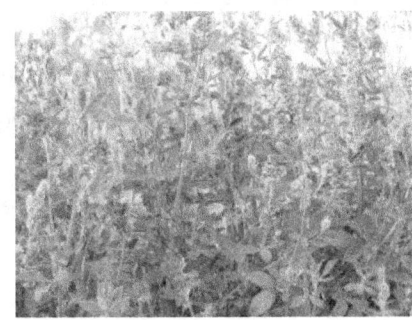

Avocado
This variety is gathered from avocado blossoms and is commonly used for dressings and sauces in food preparation. The honey is dark in color and has a rich and buttery taste.

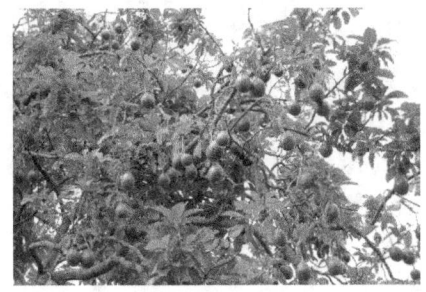

Basswood
The honey is produced from blossoms of the Basswood tree. It is light in color, delicate, and is known for its biting flavor. It is used in food preparation, as the honey works well in many recipes.

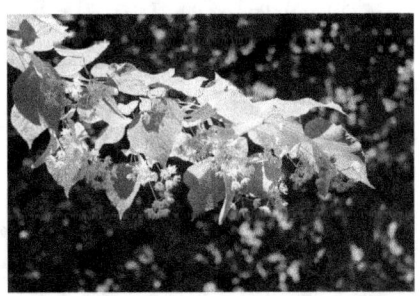

Blueberry

The honey is light amber in color and comes with a full, well-rounded flavor. The honey bees extract this nectar from the tiny white flowers of the blueberry bush. The liquid is used in preparation of baked goods and sauces.

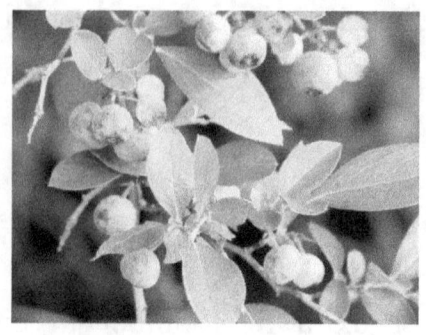

Buckwheat

Buckwheat honey is dark brown in color. The Buckwheat plants grow in cool climates and prefer light and well-drained soils. It has a strong, distinct flavor and is often used for BBQ sauces and baked goods.

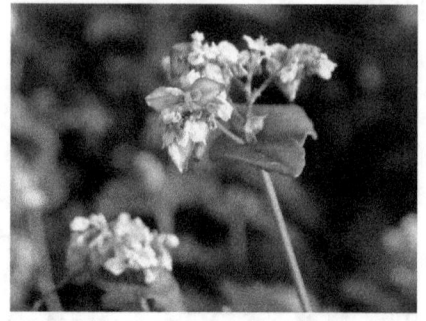

Clover

A typical honey, known for its mild taste and color and most often found on the tables at homes during meal times. Clover is known as the most common nectar producing plant, but the honey varies depending on the location and source. The color also varies based on the location from light amber to water white.

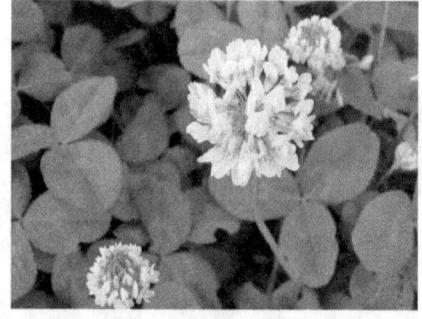

Eucalyptus

Eucalyptus honey is a rich honey extracted from the nectar of the blossoms of Eucalyptus trees, which has over 500 distinct species. The honey varies in color and flavor due to different species. It is a bold flavored honey 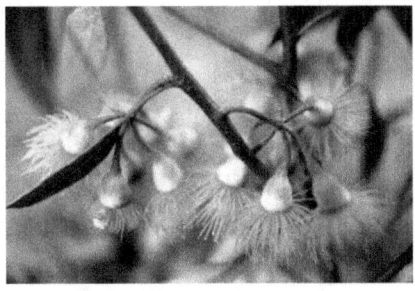 with a slightly medicinal aftertaste. This honey is ideal to be used for salad dressings, marinades, and baked goods.

Fireweed

Fireweed is a perennial herbaceous, pink flowered plant and grows in the open woods. As the name suggests, it is one of the first plants to grow in an area just after a forest fire. The trees reach up to a height of about 3-5 feet. The honey is very light in color with a delicate flavor.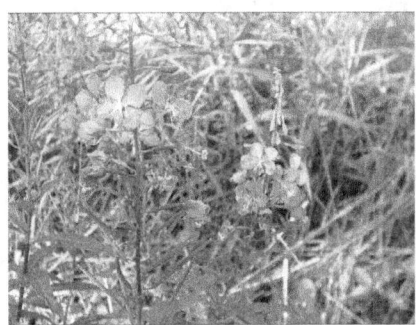

Manuka

This is the most talked about and sought after honey around the world due to its antibacterial properties. The medicinal liquid is produced from the nectar of the Manuka bush. The honey is a monofloral honey coming from New Zealand and Australia.
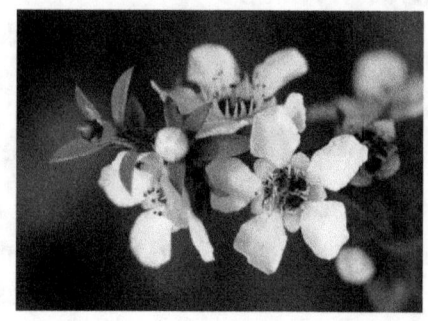
The honey is dark in color with a very strong flavor.

Orange Blossom

This honey is often a combination of citrus floral sources from Oranges and other citrus plants, such as Grapefruit or Lime. The Orange trees flower during March and April and the honey comes with a unique flavor
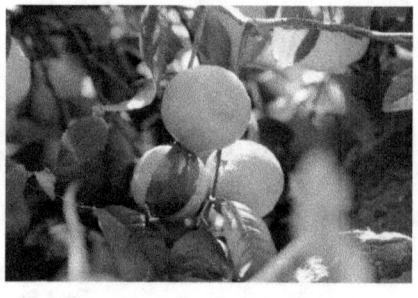
and is light amber in color. The aroma of course is of orange blossoms and the honey is often used for cakes and cookie making.

Sage

As the name suggests, sage honey comes from different species of the sage plant. The honey is light in color and is sweet in flavor. It is slow to granulate and is a favorite with honey packers for blending 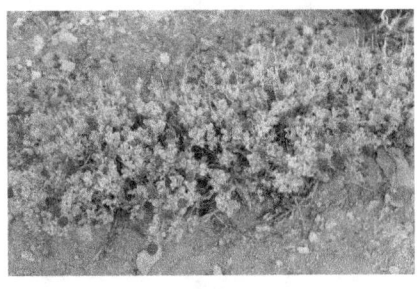 with other honeys to slow down granulation. It pairs extremely well with strong cheese.

Tupelo

This honey is taken from Tupelo trees, which have clusters of greenish flowers. The honey is light amber in color and the production season is April and May of each year. The honey is mild 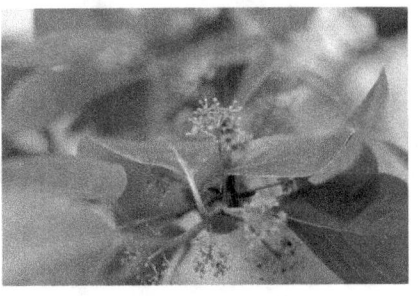 and due to high fructose content, it does not granulate.

Wildflower

Wildflower honey is also known as polyfloral honey. The honey is produced from the nectar of a variety of flowers and sometimes undefined flower sources. The flavors, aroma, and 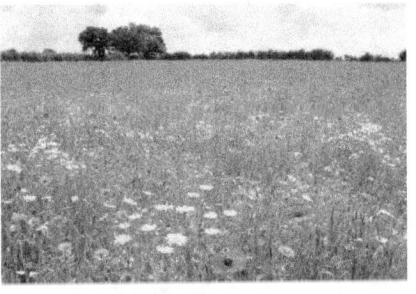 texture of the honey will vary depending from which flowers the nectar is collected, the seasons in bloom, and of course the weather conditions.

The list of varieties will go on until the flowers blossom and the little bees keep on collecting nectar from flowers all over the world.

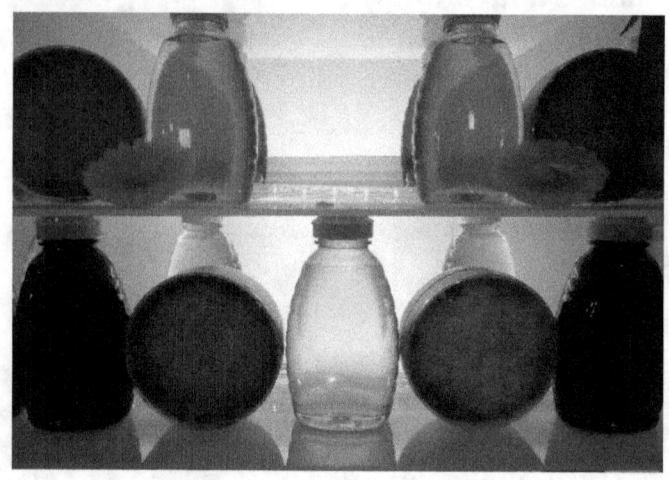

Chapter 4

What Is Raw Honey?

A natural, sweet liquid produced by the honey bees from the concentrated nectar of flowers. It is unheated, unpasteurized, unprocessed, and 100% original and differs from the average honey purchased from the grocery stores.

Raw Honey is a highly concentrated water solution of two sugars and contains many nutrients. It is full of minerals, vitamins, enzymes, and powerful antioxidants and has anti-bacterial, anti-viral, and anti-fungal properties.

Is honey Real Honey?

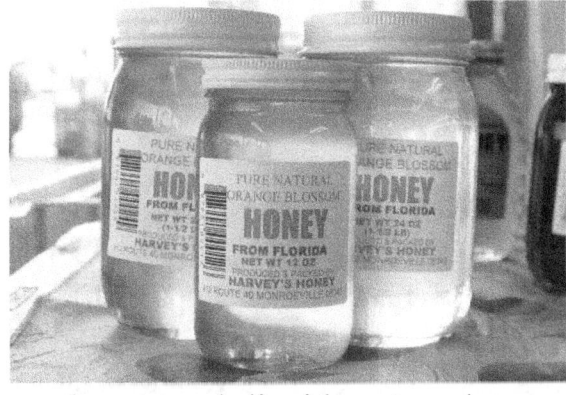

This is not true in many cases, as most honeys found in supermarkets do not contain pollen. A number of ingredients in the form of artificial sweeteners are added to the natural liquid. Any honey that constitutes these artificial components cannot be classified as raw or real honey. These artificial ingredients pose a threat to the health of the consumers and people should be vary of same.

Raw honey is often pasteurized for easy filtering and bottling so the honey bottles come out looking great and more appealing to the buyer. The pasteurization process destroys yeast cells in the honey, preventing fermentation, which causes a concern for storing honey with high moisture content for long periods. Fermentation does not pose any health issues, but it does affect the taste of honey, which is not the best.

The raw honey can be seen in different forms; liquid or solid (creamed). Raw honey in liquid form can crystalize or solidify over a period of time. It can be clear, opaque, or milky and its color can vary from white to various shades of yellow or dark colors, depending on the flower from which the bee extracts the nectar.

One cannot detect whether honey is raw or not based on the color, flavor, or form. Although some honey experts feel that they can identify raw honey by tasting, this is not the reality.

If you need to be certain that you are purchasing raw honey, it is good to look at the label on the jar of honey. If the label indicates whether the honey is pasteurized, unpasteurized, pure, etc., this would help a consumer. However, just because a label indicates the type of honey, the product cannot be guaranteed as raw honey.

In producing honey, some bee keepers do not pasteurize the honey, but heat it up to a certain degree. Heating slows down crystallization, but partially destroys the aroma, yeast, and enzymes of the honey, which are responsible for stimulating vitamins and minerals in the body.

It is always said that raw honey will have more benefits and it is often advised to consume honey from your locality rather than trying out honey coming from plants from other areas. There is belief that the local honey will help one in treating seasonal allergies and would be good for the immune system's environmental needs.

Try to source raw, organic honey, but whether it is really organic or not, no one will ever know. If the honey is organic, usually the beekeepers have to meet certain production standards and criteria. The honey cannot contain any pesticide residues or environmental pollutants. If you want the good raw honey, it is best to source from a beekeeper in the area, as you will be certain from where the honey comes from.

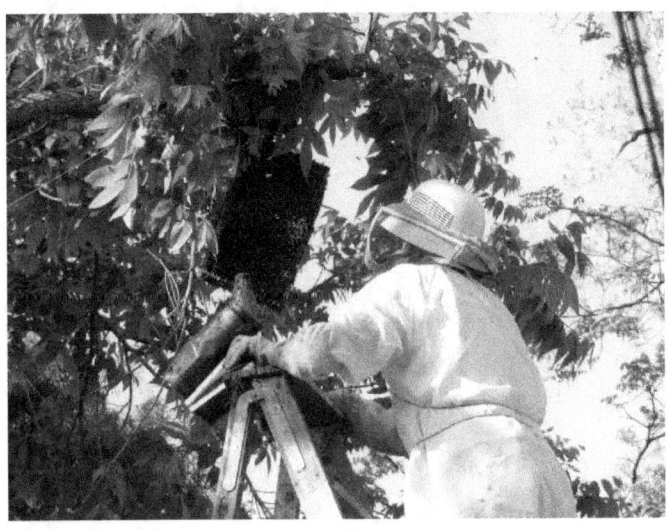

The raw honey will usually look cloudier as it contains bits and pieces of bee pollen, honeycomb remnants, propolis, bee wing fragments, etc. The real honey will granulate and crystalize to a thick formation due to its high antioxidant levels.

When hunting for raw honey available at stores, most individuals are under the misapprehension that the clearer the honey looks, the better the honey. Sadly, this is not the case, as the real honey with bits and pieces of the bees looking cloudy and smudgy is the best raw honey, which may not be commonly available for sale.

Chapter 5

The Various Forms Of Honey & Which Honey Should You Use?

Honey is a sweet golden liquid and is available in a variety of forms. Liquid honey is often laid on the table at homes, but very few have experienced the bliss of using honey in its original form as edible beeswax comb or finely crystalized, spreadable, and whipped forms.

Let us discuss a little more the different forms available.

Liquid Honey
The liquid honey is extracted from the honey comb and comes free of visible crystals. The honey is extracted by centrifugal force, gravity, or straining. This form of honey is easy to pour and mixes easily with a variety of foods. It is used for cooking and baking and if you look around, honey is most often sold in liquid form.

Comb Honey
Comb Honey is honey in its original form, straight from the honey bees' wax comb. The comb as well as the honey is edible. It is usually packaged in a variety of methods, from tiny round or square containers to entire frames directly transferred from the hives.

Cut Comb or Chunk Honey
This honey comes in liquid form and chunks of the honey comb can be found in the jar. It is also known as a liquid-cut comb blend.

Naturally Crystallized Honey
This honey is safe to eat and in this form of honey, a part of the glucose content is spontaneously crystalized.

Whipped or Creamed honey or Spun Honey
This is sold in a crystallized state. The honey is crystallized via a controlled process and at room temperature the honey can be spread like butter. This form of honey is preferred around the world over liquid honey and can be used as a substitute for jelly or jam.

What form of honey is good will be based on the consumer and it will solely depend on the purpose and of course your budget, as some forms of honey are more expensive compared to others.

Chapter 6

How To Harness Honey's Health Benefits

If one is to say honey is a remarkable substance, many will acknowledge this fact without any hesitation! With the introduction and development of different varieties of drugs and therapies to the market, the use of honey was pushed back to a forgotten corner. However, recent news articles and research indicate that the use of honey is being re-discovered and honey is becoming more important than ever before.

Research and Verdict?
A number of theories have been developed on how honey really works. The scientists are now at work trying to understand how honey helped mankind ages ago and whether we could derive the same benefits. Many believe that there was a connection between the usage of honey in the early days and its healing powers, especially on wounds.

Past records indicate that Honey has been used for medicinal purposes orally as well as topically by ancient Greeks, Egyptians, and Indians for Ayurveda and Chinese for their traditional medicine. Interestingly, a Sumerian writing in the period of 2100-2000 BC indicate honey was used as an ointment and a drug. The Greek philosopher and Scientist – Aristotle had referred to honey as "good as a salve for sore eyes and wounds". All these facts prove in no certain terms that honey was used on wounds and for other health purposes.

Remedy – How and Why?

The wounds are healed due to its antibacterial activities and the very high stickiness present in honey prevents the spread of infection. The liquid contains over 150 biologically active ingredients and the healing power is linked to its enzymes, which are added to the nectar by none other than the little bee itself. The enzymes release hydrogen peroxide (H_2O_2) and gluconic acid in one's body. H_2O_2 is a powerful antimicrobial and kills almost all germs which come into contact with it.

It is important to note that all honeys are not the same. Diverse levels of H_2O_2 can be observed in different types of honey, once again due to the various sources of nectar. Some types of honey are known as non-peroxide honey; even when the H_2O_2 activity is blocked, antibacterial effects are displayed.

Some types of honey should never be applied on an open wound whereas some honeys are so powerful that they play an important role in preventing life threatening infections.

Due to the belief and theories that honey acts as a nutrient, drug and therapy, an alternative form of treatment called Apitherapy, has been introduced in the recent years. In this treatment, honey pollen, bee bread, propolis, royal jelly, and bee venom are used for health purposes. This therapy includes replenishing energy, enhancing physical stamina, and bringing improvements to the immune system. Although there are many success stories using apitherapy, the results have yet to be proven to scientific standards and specifications.

Natural Remedy

In an era where people are looking for natural remedies, honey is regaining its popularity for a variety of reasons. It is common knowledge that honey is good for ulcers, skin infections arising from wounds and burns, bed sores, etc.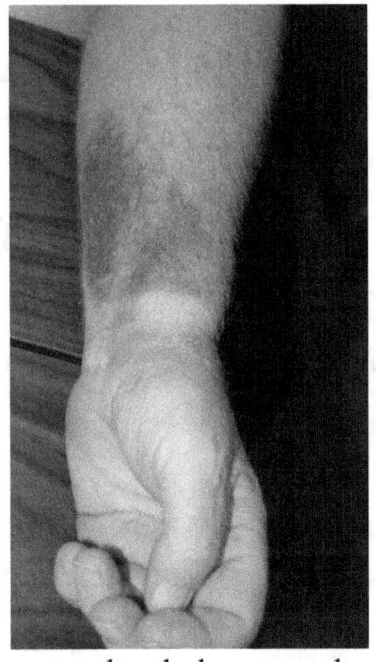

In the case of wounds, honey and its contents help the growth of new skin and tissues for speedy healing. The sugar absorbs the moisture, preventing bacteria growth and destroying the environment conducive for their survival. The sweet content in honey also helps to reduce swelling and scarring to some extent.

It is always good to use raw honey for medicinal purposes and avoid refined shop-bought honey at all costs. By applying processed honey on a wound, it is more likely that it will spread the infection and not prevent it.

In particular, medihoney and manuka honey are in demand for the treatment of wounds, burns, and ulcers. The honey applied topically creates miracles while the usually prescribed antibiotics and antiseptics remain unresponsive.

Manuka honey comes from New Zealand and is the pollen extracted from the Manuka bush, which is a medicinal plant. This honey is approved to be used for medical purposes due to its healing properties and high potency. The honey is used to overcome the following conditions.

- MRSA - Methicillin-resistant Staphylococcus Aureus

- MSSA - Methicillin-sensitive Staphylococcus Aaureus

- VRE - Vancomycin-resistant Enterococci

- Helicobacter Pylori

Honey is also often sought after as a remedy for diarrhoea, sore throat, and insomnia.

It is also important to control the use of honey in your diet. Too much of a dose might end with you being overweight and with conditions like high blood cholesterol, high blood pressure, and diabetes.

As you know, too much of anything is good for nothing!

More observations
Fresh evidence is coming into light, saying that when MediHoney dressings were applied on wounds, the patients were known to have less pain. These skin bandages have become popular due to their effectiveness on burns, skin ulcerations, scratches, scrapes, and surgical incisions. Experiments were carried out using these bandages on burns and wounds and the results were amazing, where some wounds healed completely while some showed a marked improvement.

There are so many good reasons to use honey and scrap the antibiotics. Looks like we are finally heading in the right direction with nature provided health remedies!

Ensure you have adequate stocks of honey stacked up in your home. You never know when the kids come running to you with burns, scratches, and what not.

Honey is a natural remedy for all!

Chapter 7

Nutritional Facts About Honey

Honey is goodness itself! We cannot forget the nutritional facts about honey.

As you know by now, the bees are a hive of activity and they add the enzymes to the nectar. These enzymes trigger chemical compounds, inverting sucrose into fructose and glucose. The water levels are evaporated so the honey can be kept for ages without spoiling.

Honey contains high levels of carbohydrates, fructose, and glucose and the balance of course is taken up by water, minerals, and other components as follows:

- 80% natural sugar in the form of fructose and glucose
- 18% water. The quality of honey depends on the water content and the less water content, the higher quality of honey.
- Balance 2% minerals, vitamins, protein, and contents of pollen.

Vitamins and Minerals
The vitamins can be seen in the form of B6, Thiamin, Riboflavin, Niacin, Pantothenic acid, and a few Amino acids. The mineral content found in honey consists of Calcium, Iron, Copper, Magnesium, Manganese, Phosphorus, Potassium, Sodium, and Zinc.

What a list of vitamins and minerals! Are you wondering whether or not you need anything else for your body?

The slight acid levels help to prevent the growth of germs, while its antioxidant elements help to clean up free radicals.

Since honey is a sweetener, honey can act as a substitute for sugar. However, since honey is sweeter, it is wise to use a lesser quantity. If honey is being used in a recipe instead of sugar, the liquid content of the recipe should be reduced by the same quantity.

Honey can be used for cooking and preparation of many dishes and adds its own mark to the dish in the form of flavor. Honey is also used to soften meat when used as marinades. The sweet liquid is used in savory dishes as well as cakes, biscuits, etc.

A few instances where honey can be used are listed below:

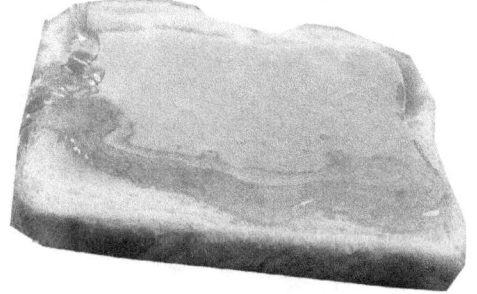

- Spread on fresh bread, toast, or a sandwich
- Add a little honey to your yoghurt
- With smoothies and juices. A little honey is great
- With tea or coffee. Reduce the sugar intake

- For pancakes, scones, crumpets, and croissants
- Puddings and cakes
- Savory dishes
- For salads, sauces, and marinades
- Most importantly, when your energy levels are down to zero, a teaspoon of honey will boost your energy levels and do the necessary.

Chapter 8

How To Harness Honey's Beauty Benefits And
Enhance Your Overall Wellness

Fact

*Honey was known to be part of Cleopatra's daily beauty
ritual.*

.If you look around you will see the array of beauty products
using honey in most of the store shelves. The advertisements
and the labels of the products carry descriptions of how
honey helps to increases your beauty, rejuvenate your skin
and also take away the stress.

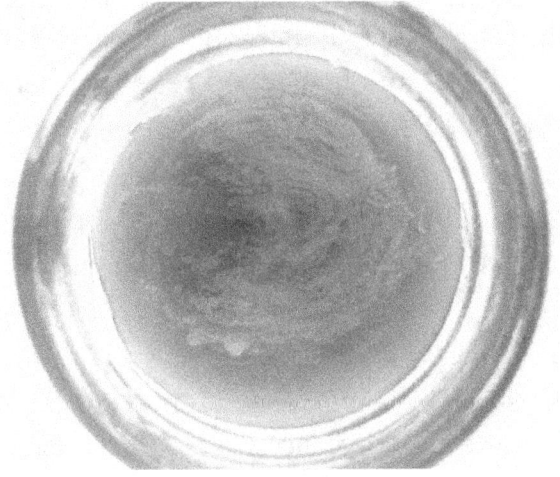

Is it true? Is honey the super power?

Looks like honey can be put to many good uses. Earlier we
talked about the health and nutrient benefits, and now on to

beauty benefits.

As much as honey was known for its healing properties, honey was also used for beauty therapy according to past records. In recent times, more and more people opt for natural ingredients in their daily beauty treatments. For whatever treatment, ensure to source quality honey instead of processed and refined brands available in the stores.

Energy booster

It is time to scrap the sugar and use honey in your food and drinks. Honey comes packed with carbohydrates providing strength and energy to our bodies and after an intake of honey, one is sure to notice the difference in energy levels.

The natural sugars prevent exhaustion and fatigue during workouts and the glucose content quickly comes to the rescue, giving the much needed energy boost and the fructose provides the sustained energy.

Research indicates that honey monitors the level of blood sugar and keeps the levels constant. What a relief!

Relaxation

If you had a stressful day, just get into your bath tub and soak away. Pour a few drops of honey into the tub and it will revitalize your aching muscles and bring about relaxation and calmness, which you are bound to enjoy. Next time, remember to take your honey jar into the bathroom.

Moisturizer

Honey acts as a moisturizer on dry skin and once applied, you can see the difference in a few days. Use honey on your parched and cracked lips and it works wonders. Rub honey on your knees and elbows just to loosen and soften them.

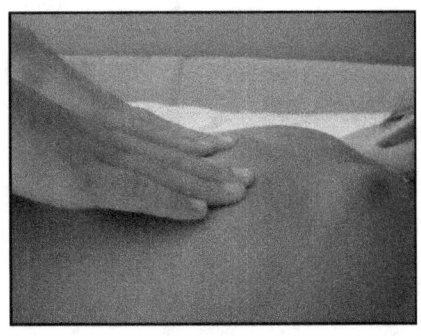

Honey can be used for facials and it will moisturize your skin and the natural contents in honey will work miracles on your skin. Honey can be used alone or you can add a little milk or sugar to make it more effective as a scrub.

Hair

Honey acts as a natural moisturizing conditioner due to its high vitamin and mineral contents. Honey is safe on the hair and ensures smooth, gleaming, and silky hair. Best use would be to add a little bit with your shampoo or you could combine it as a deep conditioning treatment. The results would be great.

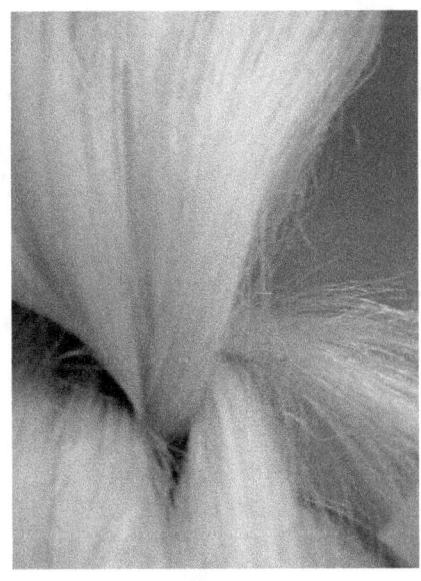

Metabolism

Hangover after Sunday evening? Just take a few spoons of honey. The fructose content in honey will raise the level of metabolism of alcohol and you will be your usual self in a few minutes.

No need to spend mints of money on expensive treatments on your body, skin, and hair. Just try nature's little secret and reap the benefits.

Fact
Honey bees communicate with each other by dancing.

Chapter 9

Delicious Honey Recipes

Enjoy these recipes made with delicious honey!

Sweet Tarts With Honey

Ingredients
1/4 cup of sugar
8 tablespoons of honey
1 (14-oz.) can of sweetened condensed milk
1 cup of milk
4 large eggs
1 large egg yolk
1/4 teaspoon of salt

Method
Preheat the oven to 350F.

Place a dash of sugar in a saucepan and cook over medium heat for about 4 minutes. Allow the sugar to melt and caramelize and add the 3 tbsp honey. Continue to stir until the mixture is smooth.

Remove from the stove and pour the warm caramelized sugar into six small bowls.

Place the sweetened condensed milk, milk, eggs, yolk, and salt in a food processor along with the balance honey and process until well blended.

Pour the mixture over sugar in each bowl. Place the little bowls in a pan with hot water up to about 1" depth. Cover with foil and bake in the preheated oven for 35 minutes. Remove from oven and allow it to cool.

Cover with a plastic wrapper and refrigerate for about 3 hours. Transfer the tarts onto a serving plate and serve.

Vanilla Honey Creams

Ingredients
1 cup of butter
2½ cups of honey
1½ cups of whipping cream
3/4 cup of brown sugar
1 teaspoon of vanilla extract
Chopped almonds or other nuts

Method
Place the butter in a saucepan and leave on the stove over medium-high temperature. Once the butter is melted, add the honey, brown sugar, and cream and blend well.

Allow the mixture to boil and continue to stir in regular intervals. Reduce the temperature and continue to cook for about 45 minutes. Remove from fire, add the vanilla extract, and mix well.

Pour into a lined tin and refrigerate till firm. Cut into pieces and sprinkle almonds or nuts on the surface. Cover each piece with plastic wrap and refrigerate up to 1 month.

Honey Glazed Spicy Chicken

Ingredients

4 tablespoons of honey
3 tablespoons of mustard
1 tablespoon of soy sauce
Freshly squeezed juice from 1 lemon
Grated zest from 1 lemon
1/4 cup of tightly packed pitted chopped prunes
1½ teaspoons of chopped fresh rosemary
1 whole roasting chicken (4 lb), trimmed of excess fat

Method

Preheat the oven to 375F.

In a bowl, mix the honey, soy sauce, and mustard and if desired, add a little water to thin the mixture.

Mix the lemon juice, prunes, zest, rosemary, and 2 tbsp of the mustard and stuff into the chicken. Place the chicken on a lined roasting pan and sprinkle the mustard mixture on the chicken.

Bake for about 50 minutes covered with foil. Take out the foil and sprinkle the balance mustard mixture on top. Bake for another 30-40 minutes until the chicken is well cooked.

Transfer the chicken to a serving tray and carve the bird when cool.

Honey Sour Rice Puddings

Ingredients

3½ ounces of long grain rice
14fl oz of <u>milk</u>
2 tablespoons of double cream
1 vanilla pod, split, seeds only
3 tablespoons of honey
1 orange peeled and sliced
1 tablespoon of honey

Method

In a saucepan, place the rice, cream, milk, honey, and vanilla seeds and bring to a boil over medium-heat. Pour into an ovenproof dish and cook in the oven for 10 minutes until the top is a golden bronze in color.

Dip the orange slices in honey and spread on top and Serve.

Honey Spicy Sauce

Ingredients

1/4 cup of mustard
1/2 cup of mayonnaise
1/4 cup of honey
1/4 teaspoon of ground red pepper
1/4 teaspoon of chili powder
1/8 teaspoon of garlic salt

Method

Place all ingredients in a bowl and mix together to form a sauce.
Serve with chicken or meat.

Bee Fun Scoops

Ingredients
1/4 cup of packed brown sugar
3/4 cup of honey
1 egg
1½ cups of flour
1/2 teaspoon of baking soda
1/2 teaspoon of salt
1/2 teaspoon of ground cinnamon

Method
Preheat the oven.

Place the butter, sugar, honey, and egg in a bowl and whisk the mixture until well blended. Add the balance ingredients and mix well.

Scoop out the mixture with a spoon and place lumps on a grease baking sheet. Bake for 10 minutes in the preheated oven to 375 degrees until light brown

Remove from the oven and allow to cool.

Serve and enjoy!

Honey Fruit Cake

Ingredients
3 cups of all-purpose flour
2¼ teaspoons of baking soda
2 teaspoons of ground cinnamon
1/2 teaspoon of salt
1/4 teaspoon of ground nutmeg
1/4 teaspoon of ground ginger
1½ cups of honey
1 cup of buttermilk
3 eggs
1/2 cup of vegetable oil
2 teaspoons of vanilla
2 cups of finely grated carrot
1 (8 ounce) can of crushed pineapple, drained
1 cup of chopped walnuts

Frosting
2 (8 ounce) packages of cream cheese, softened
1/3 cup of honey
1 teaspoon of vanilla

Method
Preheat the oven to 350 degrees.

Mix the flour, baking soda, cinnamon, salt, nutmeg, and ginger in a bowl.

In a separate bowl, mix the buttermilk, honey, eggs, oil, and a little vanilla and fold in the flour mixture. Blend well and mix the pineapple, carrots, and walnuts.

Pour the mixture into a greased baking tray and bake for 50 minutes.

For the frosting, mix all ingredients together and spread over the cake once cooled.

Honey-flavored Tiny Loaves

Ingredients
1 cup of whole-wheat flour
1 cup of flour
2 teaspoons of baking powder
1/2 teaspoon of baking soda
1/2 teaspoon of ground cinnamon
1/2 teaspoon of ground ginger
2 large eggs
1/4 cup of brown sugar
1 cup of honey
1 teaspoon of instant espresso or coffee granules stirred into
2/3 cup of hot water
1/2 cup of canola oil
1 teaspoon of vanilla extract
1 cup of coarsely chopped walnuts

Method
Preheat the oven to 350F.

Grease and flour four small loaf moulds and keep them aside.

In a bowl, mix the flours, baking soda, ginger, and cinnamon and combine well.

Beat eggs and sugar until well combined. Mix in the honey, oil, coffee and vanilla and fold in the flour mixture. Add walnuts and combine all ingredients well.

Spoon out the mixture into the loaf moulds and bake for 30 minutes. Leave to cool for a few minutes and with a knife remove the loaves gently.

Spread with butter and enjoy.

Honey Crust Bars

Ingredients
Crust
1/3 cup of unsalted butter, softened
1/3 cup of sugar
1/4 teaspoon of salt
1 cup of all-purpose flour

Filling
1/4 cup of unsalted butter
1/3 cup of sugar
1/3 cup of honey
1/2 teaspoon of vanilla
1 cup of chopped Nuts

Method
Preheat the oven to 350F.

Line a baking tray and spray with cooking spray. Place butter and sugar in a bowl and mix until well combined. Add the flour, salt, and combine until the mixture becomes crumbly.

Transfer the mixture into the baking tray and bake for 20 minutes.

Prepare the filling by mixing butter, honey, and sugar in a saucepan. Leave the saucepan on fire over medium heat and allow it to simmer for 2 minutes. Take off the stove and add the vanilla and chopped nuts.

Take out the baked crust and place the filling over the surface. Transfer to the oven and bake for another 15-20 minutes.

Allow to cool and cut into pieces.

Honeyed Chicken Tipsy Wings

Ingredients
Wings
2 tablespoons of vegetable oil + little extra
2 pounds of chicken wings, split at the joints, tips removed
2 tablespoons of unsalted butter, melted
1 teaspoon of granulated garlic
Salt and freshly ground pepper

Sauce
5 tablespoons of unsalted butter
1/3 cup of honey, plus more for drizzling
1//4 cup of chili sauce
1 tablespoon of soy sauce
2 teaspoons of fresh lime juice

Method

Preheat the oven to 350 degrees.

Grease a baking sheet with the vegetable oil. Rinse and pat dry the chicken wings with paper towels.

Place the chicken wings in a bowl.

Place 2 tbsp oil, butter, garlic with salt and pepper in a bowl and season the wings with this mixture. Place the seasoned wings on the oiled baking sheet and bake for 45 minutes until brown.

For the sauce – heat the butter until melted, add honey, sauces, and lime juice and allow the mixture to simmer. Remove from the fire and leave aside.

Transfer the baked wings into a bowl and sprinkle the warm sauce over it allowing the wings to coat well. Serve with honey and lime wedges.

Sweet Honey Slab

Ingredients
3/4 cup of white sugar
1¼ cups of honey
1/2 cup of vegetable oil
4 eggs
3 teaspoons of grated orange zest
3/4 cup of orange juice
2½ cups of plain flour
4 teaspoons of baking powder

1/4 teaspoon of baking soda
1/2 teaspoon of salt
1 teaspoon of ground cinnamon

Method
Lightly grease a pan and leave aside.

Mix the baking powder, baking soda, salt, cinnamon, and flour together and sift well.
Combine sugar, oil, eggs, honey, orange juice, and orange zest in a bowl until smooth. Fold in the flour mixture and mix well.

Pour the mixture into the prepared tin and bake in a preheated oven (350 degrees) for about 50 minutes until well baked.

Honey Nuts

Ingredients
3 tablespoons of butter, melted, plus extra for greasing the cups
2 teaspoons of clear honey, plus extra for drizzling
50 grams of self-rising flour
50 grams of ground almonds
50 grams of light muscovado sugar
1/4 teaspoon of bicarbonate of soda
2 eggs
75 Grams of Greek yogurt
1 tablespoon of pistachios, roughly chopped

Method

Lightly grease 2 cups and line the bottom with non-stick paper. Sprinkle honey on the bases.

Mix the dry ingredients together and in a separate bowl combine the butter, egg, and yogurt to a smooth paste. Combine both mixtures and pour the contents into the cups. Bake them for over 20 minutes in a preheated oven (180C) until well cooked.

Take out the little puddings using a sharp knife and place them on a serving platter. Remove the non-stick rounds and sprinkle pistachios on the surface.

Serve with ice cream or custard.

Grilled Chicken Breasts with Honey and Lime
Ingredients
2 tablespoons of butter or margarine
1 clove of chopped garlic
1 cup of honey
1½ tablespoons of lemon juice
4 skinless, boneless chicken breast halves

Method
Place the butter in a pan and allow it to melt on medium heat. Mix in the chopped garlic and cook until tender for 2 minutes. Mix in the honey and lemon juice, reserving half of the mixture for later.

Pour half of the liquid on the chicken breast halves and allow the mixture to be absorbed into the meat.

Preheat a grill, grease lightly, and place the chicken pieces on medium heat. Cook for 7 minutes per side, ensuring cooking on both sides. Baste with the honey and lemon juice and cook until the meat is brown and firm.

Honey Combo

Ingredients
1 cup of dark honey
1/3 cup of canola oil
4 cups of old-fashioned rolled oats
1 cup of unsalted pumpkin seeds
1/2 cup of cashew nuts
1/2 cup of unsalted sunflower seed kernels
2 teaspoons of sesame seeds
1 cup of dried sweetened cranberries
1 cup of chopped figs

Method
Preheat the oven to 350F.

Mix the honey and oil in a saucepan. Place on medium heat and warm for 2-3 minutes.
Add the oats, cashew nuts, and all seeds to the honey mixture and stir well. Allow the oats to be coated thoroughly.

In the meantime, prepare a lined tray and pour the mixture into the tray. Place in the oven and bake for 15 minutes.

Stir every 5 minutes and cook for another 15 minutes until golden in color.

Remove from the oven, cool, and mix in the cranberries and the figs. It can be kept stored in air tight containers.

A few useful Hints

Storage

Keep your honey bottle away from direct sunlight and store at room temperature.   Do not refrigerate under any circumstances.

If the honey crystallizes, place the bottle of honey in a pan of warm water.   Stir for a little while and the crystals will disappear.

Measuring Honey

If you need to measure honey for recipes, spray the measuring equipment with a little oil. This will ensure that the entire amount of honey will glide out of the measuring spoon or cup.

Warning!

Honey contains a few bacterial botulinum spores which come with the nectar. These spores remain unharmed during the heating/processing of honey and also are not detected by the naked eye. Due to this reason, it is advised to not give any honey to infants under the age of 18 months. These spores can grow in a baby's immature digestive system unnoticed and produce a toxin which can result in sudden death. It is best to keep processed foods containing honey away from infants as well.

Conclusion

Having come to the last page, you are now wiser to the benefits and uses of honey.

Whatever way honey is packaged- in bottles or jars, or in whichever form- liquid or comb, one can easily be convinced that honey is better than sugar.

With so many varieties to choose from- buckwheat to raw honey on supermarket shelves, you will not think twice to go for the best honey to suit your needs. Honey also retains moisture and keeps the baked food items fresh. You can use honey in almost all your dishes and it would be great to experiment and come out with your own unique honey recipe.

To sum it up, honey can be used for food, health, beauty purposes, and also as an energy booster.

Hope you enjoyed this little book. Whatever are you waiting for?
Go in and buy your wonder jar of Midas Touch – Honey!

Thank you

Other Books By Dr Brad Turner

Headache Cures Made Easy

Headaches are extremely common, especially in today's society where everyone is stressed, exhausted and forever taking on too much work. However, the big problem arises when we stop viewing headaches as something serious. Whether large or small, headaches can often be a symptom of a more severe underlying problem and ignoring them is the worst thing we can do. Whether you regularly experience primary or secondary headaches, you can use this guide to learn about the causes of headaches, the symptoms that can arise and how to tackle them if they are a common occurrence in your life. It also offers you details of natural cures, giving you useful tips and ideas to help stop that headache in its tracks, as well as information on how to prevent getting headaches and migraines in the future.

Lose Belly Fat Without Exercise

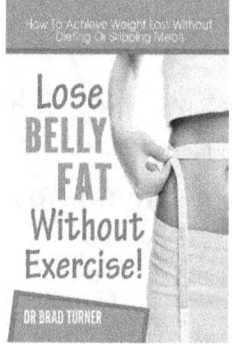

Dr Brad Turner's *Lose Belly Fat Without Exercise is* an easy to follow guide which gives you the important information you need to give you a jump start to a vibrant, radiant and sexy new you! If you are tired of counting calories, fat grams and points and or have lost your motivation with crash course Exercise programs and are tired of diets that just do not work, then this book is for you.

.

Aromatherapy The Beginner's Guide

Frankincense. Peppermint. Eucalyptus. Lemon-grass. Lavender. Who knew that these are five of the must have essential oils? Dr. Brad Turner does—and we are blessed that he's chosen to share his knowledge and expertise in his latest book, ESSENTIAL OILS. So much has been written about using oils: as cures for everything from toothaches to acne; aromatherapy and even taken internally for whatever reason is popular that day.. To our own peril, we've discovered much of this information is false. Dr. Turner gains our trust immediately with his treatise: never ingest these essential oils. And that's the beginning of an author/reader relationship that will stand the test of time…and information, because Dr. Turner tells the truth. And that's the way we like it!

The Type 2 Diabetes Cure

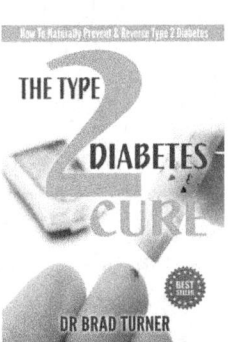

TYPE 2 DIABETES CURE just blew the myths out of the water concerning diabetes. It's the ultimate guide to diabetes, no matter the type. By defining all three types of diabetes, the author helps readers understand just how easy it is to overcome type 2 diabetes. From the sampling of mouth-watering recipes to eating plans, to exercise recommendations —TYPE 2 DIABETES CURE tells the truth--type 2 diabetes can be cured as well as prevented. And, that, my friends, is the most wonderful message in the book! Get your copy today and start your journey to incredible health.

Quit Smoking Naturally

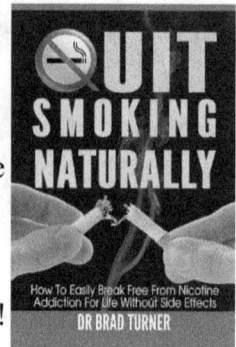

On every literary corner, there's an expert on how to quit smoking. But very few of their theories stick. Every day the weary smoker is inspired to quit, only to have his/her hopes dashed yet again. Quit Smoking Naturally is the book that may set everyone free! The genius of this book is the straightforward approach and authentic voice that provides the facts, dispels the fallacies and motivates the smoker to do what they've never done before—succeed at quitting!

Natural Antibiotics And Antivirals For Beginners

Herbal Antibiotics and Antiviral for Beginners gives a very clear description of the types and uses of medicinal herbs all over the country. This book simply reminds us about how useful the herbs were during the times of our forefathers. As the name suggests, this book is a guide on herbal antibiotics and antiviral for the beginners.

This book is a record of the various medical herbs and their properties. It also entails the preparations of the medicines from these herbs. Herbal medicines have the capacity of curing infections and diseases in the most convenient way. Not only that, but they are also almost completely harmless and have no side-effects whatsoever. The need for such medicines has become very intense since our bodies have developed a capacity to get used to the synthetic medicines.

This book specially focuses on the herbal medicinal antibiotics and antiviral. All the information given in the book has been very minutely researched and verified by professionals. So if you intend to start living by the cures of our ancestors, we suggest you order this book as soon as possible.

www.ingramcontent.com/pod-product-compliance
Lightning Source LLC
Chambersburg PA
CBHW060226290526
45789CB00003B/1435